TOP ESSENTIAL
OIL RECIPES

*The Top Essential Oil Recipes for Weight Loss,
Beauty, Anti-Aging, Natural Cleaning, Natural
Living, Natural Cures and Healthy Lifestyles*

JOY LOUIS

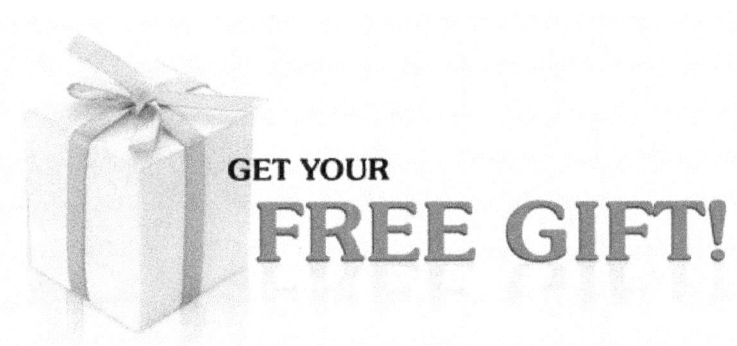

GET YOUR

FREE GIFT!

WAIT! BEFORE YOU CONTINUE – DO YOU LIKE FREE BOOKS?

My **FREE Gift** to You!! As a way to say **Thank You** for downloading my book, I'd like to offer you more **FREE BOOKS**! Each time we release a NEW book, we offer it first to a small number of people as a test–drive. Because of your commitment here in downloading my book, I'd love for you to be a part of this group. You can join easily here→ **http://joylouisbooks.com/**

Do You Enjoy **FREE BOOKS**? Do you like books that are Life Changing, Inspirational, Motivational and Informative? We **LOVE** sharing **FREE BOOKS** with people like you. It's easy to join just by clicking here→ http://joylouisbooks.com/

BEFORE CONTINUING – FREE BOOKS!
From the Author Joy Louis

Table of Contents

From Author Joy Louis:

I'm so very excited and honored that you've picked up this book and want to learn more about essential oils!

Before you read on and really dive into the book let me introduce myself…

My name is Joy, and I'm an all Natural-Organic-Homemade "Everything" Person. In other words: I have a natural solution for pretty much everything in my life!

My "all natural" way of living started a few years back when I was sick and tired of being sick, FAT and tired. I was eating pretty healthy (or so I thought): I ate peanut butter jelly sandwiches for lunch every day, snacked on cereal protein bars in between meals (these are healthy, right?) and drank Diet Coke (because isn't Diet Coke better than sugar? No calories versus a mother lode of sugar that would go straight to my butt. I'll take the "no sugar" please and thank you). However, despite living my so-called "healthy" lifestyle, I kept gaining weight, and lost all energy and motivation to do anything; I even started to dread taking my dearest Pretzel (my sweet dog of 7 years) out for her daily walk around the neighborhood!

That's when I knew I'd had enough. I decided to start searching for a better way; a way that has now proven to give me more energy than I ever imagined possible and also helped me lose 45 pounds of stubborn body fat in the process. I made a drastic change, 180-degree turn in all my habits.

So here it is. My so called "secret, hidden formula" I used to get to where I am today is: I went ALL NATURAL. Not a very sexy answer, is it? Well I have to tell you, a lot of times we complicate things way too much when looking for an answer. More often than not the solution to our problems is very simple. However... simple doesn't mean it's easy - far from it!

As for me, I don't know how I gathered the willpower to do this, but somehow I managed to throw out all of my garbage foods (i.e cereal bars, cookies, chips and so on) and replaced them with organic, GMO-free vegetables, fruits and lean meats all within one day. I completely went cold turkey: I stopped using all of the popular soaps and lotions out there that are FILLED with toxins, and instead I made my own, or found other safe brands and options. A short time after my big lifestyle change I learned about essential oils, and soon they became a necessity in my every day life. They are such an important part of my life and have helped me so much that I have now written a book about them. The world needs to know about these oils, their healing properties and the overall well-being of the people who use them!

As for myself, I use them in almost everything. They're my go-to problem solver, my all-natural medicine cabinet. No more artificial pain killers or medicine with a hundred possible side effects. Essential oils keep my food cravings in check, clear out my sinuses when feel a cold coming on, straighten out the wrinkles and lines coming on in my face, and uplifts my mood the days I feel anxious. For the first time in my life, I can finally say I feel 100% present and alive! I have started to love my body and I have found a true passion in helping others, hence why I decided to write this book. I truly hope you find this book helpful, and please let me know if you have any questions about any of the content.

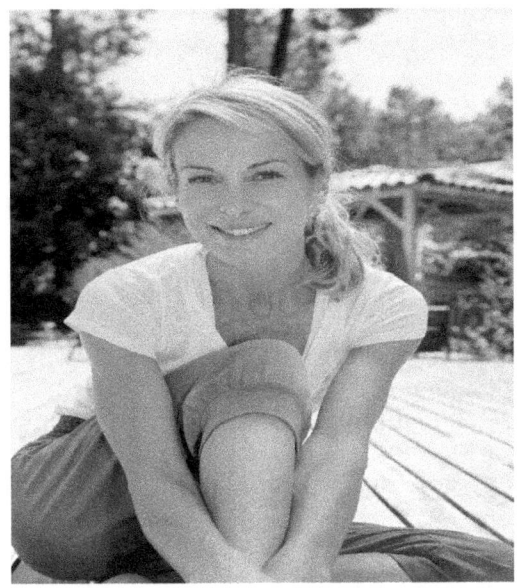

With much love,

Joy Louis
Connect with Joy here:
https://www.facebook.com/JoyLouisBooks

SEE MORE OF JOY'S BOOKS HERE:
https://www.amazon.com/author/joylouis

Balance your Life with Essential Oil Recipes

Recently I visited an essential lavender farm in Central Utah. I learned that essential oils are those wonderful and highly concentrated plant ingredients that have potent medicinal and high cosmetic qualities. Essential oils are considered the life force of the plant and nature's living energy. Essential oils are high in antibacterial, antiviral, and antifungal properties. They are excellent in homemade cleaning recipes, support for traditional medications, bug repellents, inhalation, and massage. Essential oils are miniscule in molecular size that gives them a unique property that can be absorbed into the skin. Their molecule size makes them the ingredient perfect for personal care items that heal, soften and nourish.

You will never see a patented essential oil. They are totally natural and will never be used as a prescription drug or manufactured artificially. It does take an astronomical number of bits and parts of the plant to make essential oils. Lavender takes 200 pounds of plant material to make on pound of essential. Over

1000 pounds of rose petals to make one pound of rose essential oil. Have you ever held a lavender flower or a rose petal? Gives you an interesting perspective on how many flowers and petals it takes to make a very little amount of essential oil.

If you want a truly wonderful essential oil experience, walk through a lavender "farm" at the height of blooming. The smells are healing and the plants themselves are gorgeous. Just watch out for the bees who love to flit around from flower to flower.

What makes essential oils so believable is their history. Historically essential oils were the foundation of beauty, health and balance. The Bible recognizes at least 200 references to aromatics, incense and ointments. Five thousand years ago ancient medical practitioners used essential oils for treating the sick and anointing the emotionally compromised. Today you can find essential oils used in aromatherapy, massage, emotional health, nutritional supplements, personal care products, household recipes and so much more. Personally, I could not live without my supply of essential oils.

These awesome essential oil recipes for beauty come from nature's treasure trove of elements to help you feel well inside and out.

Being a natural beauty is no mean feat, but being beautiful naturally is very easy to do. Love the essential oil recipes for beauty. Not only are they good for you, but essential oil blends give you a head start on staying balanced and beautiful. If you are tired of the advertisements that "claim" you can get younger skin with their chemical products (and I have tried them all), do something that really works; start with what's inside and work to the outside.

Essential oils have the most wonderful benefits for the skin. Just about any skin condition from acne to aging, dryness to illness and everything in between can benefit from essential oils. Combine with the right carrier oils and you will see spectacular results.

Top 10 Essential Oils for Skincare

- Lavender essential is an oil I suggest you keep in your medicine, beauty, cooking, well just about everything, cabinet. Lavender helps you relax and gives you a mechanism to adapt to stress. Lavender regenerates skin cells, helps hydrate mature skin, and lessens the appearance of sun spots and scarring. I personally could not live without my lavender essential oil.

- Carrot seed essential oil help to smooth skin and assists with cell regeneration. It does fade scars and improves the toning of aging skin. I can attest to this! As the years go by I find that my skin is less elastic and doesn't "snap" back as easy after a day in the sun. Carrot seed essential oil brings back that elasticity.

- Lemon essential oil is a natural astringent and is also antibacterial. It is beneficial if you have oily and acne-prone skin. It tones the skin and reduces the appearance or pores. Lemon essential oil is one of the better known essential oils and is prized for its stimulating, anti-infection, detoxifying, and antiseptic properties.

- Geranium essential oil regulates oil produced in the skin and reduces acne. Geranium oil improves skin elasticity and tightens the skin which helps to reduce the appearance of wrinkles. It also helps heal bruises, broken capillaries, burns, eczema and other skin conditions.

- Frankincense essential oil is a must for antibacterial and anti-inflammatory benefits. It is a natural toners and helps even out skin tones. Frankincense protects existing skin cells and encourages new cell growth. Wrinkles are reduced, tightened skin is a plus and it soothes dry skin.

- Ylang-ylang essential oil is a particular favorite of mine. It has a floral fragrance that is rich with scent. It controls oil production and minimizes breakouts. Ylang-ylang regenerates skin cells and smooths fine lines.

- Patchouli essential oil is amazing for aging skin. New cell growth is promoted by patchouli and the appearance of fine line and wrinkles seem to disappear. It is also an antiseptic, antifungal and has antibacterial properties and the smell brings you down to earth.

- Myrrh essential oil is my love. It benefits aging skin and has strong anti-inflammatory properties that help improve skin elasticity. Again, myrrh is an oil that reduces the appearance of fine lines and wrinkles.

- Neroli essential oil is a wonder if you have oily and mature skin. Fine lines seem to disappear with neroli and sagging skin is toned. There is a chemical called citral in neroli that regenerates cells. It helps and prevents stretch marks. I rub neroli on the stretch marks on my hips and these unsightly marks just seem, to me, to melt.

- Tea Tree essential oil is a well-known essential oil for acne-prone skin. It has great antibacterial properties that ward off bacteria. Oil production regulating properties in tea tree oil will decrease the incidence of acne breakouts. I could have used tea tree oils when I was a teenager!

- Always mix these oils in a carrier oil to a maximum of 5%. In other words, to 1 ml of carrier oil, you add 1 drop of essential oil. Do a patch tests on your inner forearm to make sure your skin does not react adversely to the oils.

Conversions when Blending Essential Oils

Size Conversions:

- 3 teaspoons (tsp) = 1 tablespoon (tbsp.)

- 2 tablespoons (tbsp.) = 1 ounce (oz.)

- 6 teaspoons (tsp) = 1 ounce (oz.)

- 10 milliliter (ml) = 1/3 oz. or 2 teaspoons.

- 15 milliliter (ml) = 1/2 oz.

- 30 milliliter (ml) = 1 oz. or 2 tablespoons

- 10 milliliter (ml) = approximately 300 drops

Chapter 1

PERSONAL CARE

Essential oils have been used in personal care products for thousands of years. Ancient Egyptians used essential oils to nourish the skin and hair and enhance the complexion. Essential oils were mixed into kohl to keep it pure. These natural oils will do the same for you.

Natural essential oils also promote the general health and balance of your body.

I would never put any product on my face that did not contain the nourishing properties of essential oils. Once you have tried some of these recipes, you won't go back to store-bought products.

Lip Balm

Ingredients

- 1 tablespoon Organic Shea Butter

- 3 tablespoons Sunflower Oil Almond or Grapeseed Oils

- 1 tablespoon + 1 teaspoon Beeswax

- 25 drops organic Sweet Orange essential oil

- 5 drops Organic Clove essential oil

Instructions

- Melt the beeswax and Shea butter. Stir in all the other ingredients (essential oils). Pour into a jar and allow to harden.

Skin Care

Dry Skin Reliever

Ingredients

- 1 tablespoon Rosehip oil

- 1 tablespoon Jojoba oil

- 2 tablespoons Avocado oil

- 6 drops of Jasmine Essential Oil

- 5 drops Sandalwood Essential Oil

- 6 drops of Ylang-Ylang Essential Oils

Instructions

- Thoroughly add the carrier oils and essential oils to a small, dark, glass bottle. Apply two to three drops to face and neck on a daily basis.

Normal or Sensitive Skin Serum

Ingredients

- 1 tablespoon Rose Hip Seed oil

- 2 tablespoons Apricot Kernel Oil

- 12 drops of Ylang-Ylang Essential Oil

- 18 drops of Chamomile Essential oil

Instructions

- Add the carrier and essential oils to a small dark glass bottle. Shake well. Use two to three drops to face and neck once a day.

Anti-Aging Face Serum

Ingredients

- 2 teaspoons Carrot Oil

- 1 tablespoon Rose Hip Seed oil

- 2 tablespoons Apricot Kernel oil

- 16 drops Frankincense Essential oil

- 16 drops Rose Essential oil

- 8 drops Neroli Essential oil

Instructions

- Mix the carrier and essential oils in a small dark glass bottle. Use two to three drops to face and neck once a day.

Nourishing Face Serum Recipe

Ingredients

- 3 tablespoons Almond oil

- 5 drops of Chamomile Essential oil

- 10 drops Neroli Essential oil

Instructions

- Mix the carrier and essential oils in a small dark glass bottle. Use two to three drops on face and neck once a day.

Wrinkle Prevention for a 40s Skin

Ingredients

- 2 drops Rosemary essential oil

- 2 drops Lemon essential oil

- 10 drops Carrot essential oil

- 10 drops Evening Primrose essential oil

- 10 drops Fennel essential oil

- 10 drops Neroli essential oil

- 10 drops Lavender essential oil

- 3 tablespoons Apricot oil, Almond oil OR Hazelnut oil

Instructions

- Mix the carrier and essential oils in a small dark glass bottle. Use two to three drops to face and neck once a day.

Anti-Aging Face Serum

Ingredients

- 1 tablespoon Jojoba Oil

- 2 teaspoons Rosehip Oil

- 2 teaspoons Calendula Oil

- 1 teaspoon Wheat germ Oil

- 4 drops Rosewood Essential oil

- 4 drops Rose Otto Essential oil

- 4 drops Lavender Essential oil

Instructions

- Mix the carrier and essential oils in a small dark glass bottle. Use two to three drops to face and neck once a day.

Vitamin E Face Serum

Ingredients

- 3 drops Roman Chamomile Essential oil

- 2 drops Bergamot Essential oil

- 5 drops Lavender Essential oil

- 3 tablespoon Jojoba Oil

- 1 tablespoon Grapeseed Oil

- 1/2 teaspoon Vitamin E Oil

Instructions

- Mix the carrier and essential oils in a small dark glass bottle. Use two to three drops to face and neck once a day.

Facial Scrubs & Exfoliator
Epsom Exfoliate

Ingredients

- 2 cups of Epsom Salt

- 1/4 cup of Petroleum jelly

- 3 drops of Lavender essential oil.

Instructions

- Mix ingredients. Pour into a glass jar and use the mixture to gently scrub away dry skin patches.

Face Cleanser with Almond Oil

Ingredients

- 6 tablespoons Sweet almond oil

- 1/4 cup ground almonds

- 1 1/2 tablespoons apple cider vinegar

- 1 1/2 tablespoons water

- 6 drops essential oil of your choice

Instructions

- Blend into a smooth paste. Add more water if too thick. Store in a glass jar in the refrigerator. This blend can last for up to three weeks.

Face Cleanser with Cocoa Butter

Ingredients

- 6 tablespoons Cocoa butter

- 2 1/2 tablespoons Grapeseed oil

- 2 1/2 tablespoons water

- 5 drops Sandalwood

- 1 tablespoon Brown sugar PER wash

Instructions

- Melt cocoa butter in a microwave. Add in the water and grapeseed oil. Whisk until room temperature than add essential oils. Store in a dark, glass jar. Add brown sugar to your hands just before washing your face.

Face Cleanser — For Gentle Use

Ingredients

- 6 tablespoon of each: sweet almond, jojoba, and grapeseed oils.

- 9 drops Bergamot essential oils

- 9 drops Rose essential oils

- 6 drops Lavender essential oils

- 1 tablespoon Brown sugar PER wash

Instructions

- Add carrier and essential oils to a dark glass bottle. Shake gently to blend. Store in a dark, glass bottle in a cool place. Add brown sugar to hands and wash your face. Apply a small amount of oil recipe to face and massage to cleanse. Rinse with warm water and a wash cloth. Produces super silky skin.

Lavender Face Cleanser Recipe

This is the perfect recipe to clean and add antibiotic properties to your face. Gets rid of that sticky feeling you sometime have when you wear makeup.

Ingredients

- 6 tablespoon Grape seed oil

- 10 drops of Lavender essential oil

- 5 drops of Geranium essential oils

- 5 drops of Rose essential oils

- 1 tablespoon Brown sugar PER wash

Instructions

- Add carrier and essential oils to a dark glass bottle. Shake gently to blend. Store in a dark, glass bottle in a cool place. Add brown sugar to hands and wash your face. Apply a small amount of oil recipe to face and massage to cleanse. Rinse with warm water and a wash cloth. Produces super silky skin

Face Scrub with Oatmeal and Almond

Oatmeal soothes and cleans and is a very nice non-alkaline soap substitute. If your skin is dry, use ground almonds. Almonds are natural moisturizing cleansers.

Ingredients

- 1 part ground oatmeal or ground almonds

- 3 to 5 drops of essential oil of choice

Instructions

- Use a blender to mix all ingredients. Scrub face with preparation at night. Pat dry.

Lotions, Creams and Body Oils
Mango Butter Cream for Anti-Aging

One of my favorite creams is almost good enough to eat!

Ingredients

- 2 Tbs. Beeswax

- 2 Tbs. Mango butter

- 8 Tbs. Coconut oil

- 10 drops Carrot seed essential oil

Instructions

- Melt wax and butter together. Add coconut oil. Stir well and allow to cool. Once cool, add essential oils. Mix until smooth. Pour into jar and allow to harden. (Mango butter reduces degeneration of skin cells and restores elasticity).

Homemade Lotion with Essential Oils

This hand lotion recipe has a very nice smell and is very soothing to hands that are overworked. I use this lotion all the time.

Ingredients

- 2 oz. Beeswax

- 8 oz. Jojoba oil

- 10 drops Carrot seed essential oil

- 10 drops Myrrh

- 10 drops Frankincense

- 10 drops Lavender

Instructions

- Melt first two ingredients together. Blend thoroughly and let cool to room temperature. Add essential oils, pour into a dark glass jar and cool completely.

- Take this oil with you to the beach. The carrot essential oil adds hydration and help get rid of wrinkles, and the myrrh is perfect as an astringent.

Grapeseed Body Oil

Ingredients

- 4 teaspoons Cranberry Oil

- 4 teaspoons Pomegranate Oil

- 4 tablespoon Grapeseed Oil

- 15 drops Carrot Essential oil

- 10 drops Myrrh Essential oil

- 10 drops Neroli Essential oil

Instructions

- Add the carrier oils to a dark, glass jar. Mix in the essential oils. Before each use, shake well.

Eczema Cream Lotion Recipe

I do not suffer from eczema, but my best friend does. She uses this essential oil recipe to look and feel great.

Ingredients

- 1 tablespoon Beeswax

- 2 oz. Shea Butter

- 2 tablespoons Sweet Almond oil

- 10 drops German Chamomile

- 10 drops Lavender

- 10 drops Vitamin E oil

Instructions

- Melt beeswax and shea butter in a double boiler until liquefied. Mix together thoroughly. Allow to come to room temperature, add essentials. Cool completely before using.

Lavender Body Oil Recipe

Ingredients

- 4 oz. Macadamia Nut Oil

- 10 drops Chamomile Roman Essential Oil

- 10 drops Lavender Essential Oil

- 10 drops Bergamot Essential Oil

Instructions

- Combine the essential oil to the carrier oils in a dark glass bottle.

Psoriasis Body Oil Recipe

Ingredients

- 3 oz. Apricot Kernel Oil

- 1 oz. Pomegranate Oil

- 10 drops Bergamot Essential Oil

- 10 drops Helichrysum Essential Oil

Instructions

- Mix carrier and essential oils in a dark, glass bottle. Shake well.

Rose Geranium Body Oil Recipe

Ingredients

- 4 oz. Apricot Kernel Oil

- 10 drops Geranium Essential Oil

- 10 drops Rose Essential Oil

- 10 drops Bergamot Essential Oil

Instructions

- Mix carrier and essential oils in a dark, glass bottle. Shake well.

Eye Preparations

Anti-Aging Eye Restorative

Ingredients

- 1 ounce Jojoba oil

- 5 drops Chamomile essential oil

- 5 drops Rose essential oil

Instructions

- Combine jojoba oil and essential oils in a dark glass bottle that has a dropper top. Use 1 drop of the mixture to your finger and gently smooth the oil beneath your eye. Work onto the area just beneath your brow bone. Avoid getting oil on your eyelids.

Lavender Eye Serum

Ingredients

- 3 Tbs. Jojoba oil

- 1 Tbs. Grape seed oil

- 5 drops Lavender Essential Oil

- 3 drops Roman chamomile Essential Oil

- 2 drops Bergamot Essential Oil

Instructions

- Mix all these oils in a glass eye dropper jar. Shake well. Take one drop and gently apply to eye area. This can also be used as an allover facial serum once a night.

Eye Wrinkle Cream Recipe

Ingredients

- 3 tsp. Jojoba oil

- 3 tsp. Apricot-kernel oil

- 1 tsp. Cranberry Seed Oil

- 1 tsp. Beeswax

- 5 drops Carrot-seed essential oil

Instructions

- Melt beeswax and carrier oils in a heavy saucepan. Stir while mixture cools to room temperature. Add carrot seed essential to mixture and pour into a dark, glass bottle. Smooth the mixture around your eye before you go to bed. Use just a tiny drop; a little goes a long way.

Aloe Vera Eye Cream

Ingredients

- 1 teaspoon Apricot Kernel oil

- 1 teaspoon Grapefruit essential oil

- 1 teaspoon grated Beeswax

- 1/2 teaspoon Aloe Vera gel

- 1 Vitamin E capsule

Instructions

- Melt oils and butter in a double boiler. After wax has melted, remove from heat. Use a wooden spoon and stir in aloe vera. Cool to room temperature and add grapefruit essential oil and vitamin E (puncture the capsule and squeeze out its contents), stir well. Pour into a small glass jar, cool, and tightly seal. Use before going to bed.

Lavender Eye Recipe

As with any recipe that calls for lavender, you will feel rejuvenated and the lavender oil is an antiseptic.

Ingredients

- 3 Tbs. Jojoba oil

- 1 Tbs. Grape seed oil

- 5 drops Lavender Essential Oil

- 3 drops Roman chamomile Essential Oil

- 2 drops Bergamot Essential Oil

Instructions

- Mix ingredients in a dark, glass bottle with and eye dropper. Shake well before using and apply one drop to the eye area before you go to bed. You can also use this all over your face.

Anti-Wrinkle Eye Serum for the Younger Woman

Ingredients

- 2 tablespoons Hazelnut oil

- 15 drops Jojoba oil

- 3 drop Lavender essential oil

- 3 drop Rosewood essential oil

- 9 drops Carrot essential oil

- 2 capsules Vitamin E

Instructions

- Mix all oils in a glass eye dropper jar. Shake well before you use and apply one drop to eye areas before bedtime.

Vitamin E Eye Serum Recipe

Vitamin E is a well-known anti-aging vitamin. Use this recipe often to keep those wrinkles away from your eyes!

Ingredients

- 2 tablespoons Hazelnut oil

- 6 drops Borage seed oil

- 9 drops Evening primrose oil

- 6 drops Lavender essential oil

- 6 drops Carrot essential oil

- 2 capsule Vitamin E

Instructions

Mix all oils in a glass eye dropper jar. Shake well and apply one drop to eye area before bedtime.

Anti-Aging Eye Serum Recipe

Ingredients

- 2 tablespoons Hazelnut oil

- 6 drops Borage seed oil

- 3 drop Chamomile German essential oil

- 3 drop Carrot oil essential oil

Instructions

Use a dark glass eye dropper bottle. Shake well before each use. Apply one drop to eye area before bedtime.

Bath Time

Essential oils are the most awesome additives you your bath water. However, when using essential oils in baths, do not apply to running bath water or the oil will evaporate. Add essential oils with a carrier oil to dilute and for a more enjoyable bath soak. Jojoba and sweet almond oils are perfect for bathing. Just use 1 tablespoon carrier oil with your oils. Avoid using essential oils on children or while pregnant. Essential oils do come with warning labels and instructions; do read these!

Detox Bath

Ingredients

- 1 Tablespoon of dry mustard and cayenne pepper

- 5 drops each of ginger essential and cypress oil

Instructions

- Mix ingredients in a glass of water. Stir into tub of very hot water. Before getting into the tub squeeze 2 lemons into 60 oz. of cool water and add 9 drops of lemon or orange essential oils, and 6 drops of cypress essential oil. Drink 20 oz. before getting into the bath. Soak for about 20 minutes and drink another 20 oz. of water while in the tub. When you get out of the tub, immediately wrap yourself in the frozen sheet for up to 15 minutes. Drink the remaining 20 oz. of water. You can also take a capsule of grapefruit essential oil before jumping into the tub.

Feeling Awful Bath Soak

Ingredients

- Two cups Epsom Salt

- 3 drops eucalyptus essential oil

- 3 drops rosemary essential oil

Instructions

- Combine all ingredients and pour into the water as your tub fills. Epsom salts contain magnesium that will ease stress, lower blood pressure, create a relaxed feeling and raise energy levels. If you experience migraine headaches, this "Feeling Awful Bath Soak", will definitely help you. Epson salts and essential oils will also help to reduce inflammation, plus relieve pain and muscle cramps.

Bath Bombs

Ingredients

- 1/2 cup baking soda

- 1/4 cup citric acid

- 1/4 cup cornstarch

- 2 tablespoons sweet almond oil

- 1 teaspoon water

- 1 teaspoon essential oil (your favorite scent – mine is peppermint)

- 1/8 teaspoon borax

Instructions

- Mix the first 3 ingredients together. Combine oil, water, essential oil and borax in a separate bowl. Add liquid to dry ingredients a small amount at a time and mix with a pastry blender. Roll into balls. Cure overnight to dry. Store in a glass jar.

Milk Bath

This recipe represents the ultimate in luxury. I get the water as hot as I can stand it, take in my favorite book, and lock the bathroom door.

Ingredients

- 1 1/2 cups buttermilk

- 3 tablespoons Epsom salts

- 1 tablespoon Olive oil

- 3 drops Lavender essential oil

Instructions

- Simply combine ingredients and pour as your tub fills.

Lavender& Honey Milk Bath

Ingredients

- 10 drops Lavender Essential oil

- 1 1/2 cups whole milk

- 1/3 cup Honey

Instructions

- Mix all ingredients in a bowl, pour into a jar, and shake before you use. Store in the refrigerator for up to one week.

Bath Cookies

Ingredients

- 2 cups finely ground sea salt

- 1/2 cup baking soda

- 1/2 cup cornstarch

- 2 T light oil

- 1 tsp vitamin E oil

- 2 eggs

- 5-6 drops essential oil of your choice

Instructions

- Preheat oven to 350° F. Combine ingredients and form into a dough. Form dough into one teaspoon-sized balls, and gently place them on a non-greased cookie sheet. Sprinkle the bath balls with herbs, flower petals, cloves, or citrus zest. Bake for ten minutes or until lightly browned. Allow cookies to completely cool and drop into a warm bath.

ROMAN BATH SOAK

This is a wonderful and very indulgent bath soak ideal for a cold winter day.

Ingredients

- 1 cup of sesame, olive, apricot or avocado oil

- 1 cup of mild shampoo or liquid Castile soap

- 1/2 tsp. of your favorite essential oil

Instructions

- Combine all ingredients in a decorate jar or bottle with a lid. Shake before each use, and pour one to two tablespoons into your running bath water. The mild shampoo will emulsify and disburse the oil throughout the bath water.

PSORIASIS Bath Salts

Ingredients

- 2 C Epsom Salts

- 1 C Sea Salt or Rock Salt

- 2 tablespoon Baking Soda

- 3 drops Lavender essential oil

- 3 drops Sandalwood essential oil

- 3 drops German chamomile essential oil

Instructions

- Mix salts together in a bowl and stir in remaining ingredients. Add one drop of essential oil at a time and continue stirring. Allow mixture to dry for about six hours. Store in glass jars.

Itch Reliever Bath Salts

I personally use this for dry and itchy winter skin. It really works!

Ingredients

1 cup Sea Salt or Rock Salt

2 tablespoon Baking Soda

3 drops Jasmine essential oil

3 drops Peppermint essential oil

3 drops Lavender essential oil

Instructions

Mix salt together in a bowl and stir in remaining ingredients. Add one drop of essential oil at a time and continue stirring. Allow mixture to dry for about six hours. Store in glass jars.

Chapter 2

ESSENTIAL OILS AND WEIGHT LOSS

S melling your way to losing weight may sound kinky, but according to research in Japan, there are definitely certain scents that trigger weight loss. The essential oil fairy is not going to come out and tap you on the shoulder and you automatically lose weight, but aromatherapy weight loss remedies manage cravings and address stress, depression and anxiety that can lead to overeating.

When you inhale an essential oil the microscopic molecules affect a part of your brain called the hypothalamus. The hypothalamus contains a satiety center that controls feeling hunger and fullness. Certain essential oil molecules will send a signal to the hypothalamus that you are full.

Essential oils can balance your appetite and help relieve food cravings, enhance digestion and metabolism and burn excess fat.

Use the scent of essential oils to make your brain think you have eaten enough. You will feel full, and you will eat less. Give it a try and be pleasantly surprised.

Inhalation

Use this handy aromatherapy inhaler when you feel cravings. Take three long and slow deep breaths of the aroma. Take a break for a moment, then take three more deep breaths. Flood your nose with scent. It really does work, and you won't lose out on the satisfaction of eating what you love.

Pour a teaspoon of coarse sea salt in a dark glass bottle and add one of these blends:

Weight Loss Citrus Blend

- 30 drops Grapefruit essential oil

- 4 drops Lemon essential oil

- 1 drop Ylang-Ylang essential oil

Weight Loss Mint Blend

- 20 drops Peppermint essential oil

- 10 drops Bergamot essential oil

- 4 drops Spearmint essential oil

- 1 drop Ylang-Ylang essential oil

Weight Loss Herbal Blend

- 15 drops Basil essential oil

- 15 drops Marjoram essential oil

- 1 drop Oregano essential oil

- 1 drop Thyme essential oil

Body Wrap

Drinking water helps with fat burn. This is something I have done at a party with a group of fun friends. We did laugh a lot and take pictures, which are hidden away in a safe!

Ingredients

- 15 drops of Grapefruit essential oil

- 10 drops of Lemongrass essential oil

- 10 drops of Cypress essential oil

- 10 drops of Lemon essential oil

- High quality carrier oil

Instructions

- Mix all ingredients together and rub all over your body from your rib cage down to your knees. Wrap your body in saran or any type of plastic wrap. Wrap blankets, towels or quilts around your body to maintain body heat. Leave on for one hour. Drink plenty of water and use organic lemons or one drop of lemon essential oil per every 8 oz. of water. Drink as much water as you can.

Cellulite Baths

Fill the tub with warm water. Add a cup of apple cider vinegar. Mix one recipe of these essential oils in a separate bottle. Jump in your bath and begin adding the essential oils. Swish them around in the water. Soak for approximately 30 minutes. Add a few drops of olive oil to the water if your skin tingles or burns.

Possible Blends for Cellulite Baths

- 5 drops of Citronella

- 5 drops of sandalwood

- 5 drops of grapefruit

- 5 drops of Orange essential oil

- 5 drops of Amyris

- 5 drop of Tasmanian lavender essential oil

- 5 drops of Ginger essential oil

- 5 drops of cypress essential oil

- 5 drops of Lemon essential oil

- 5 drops of Sweet fennel essential oil

- 5 drops of Geranium essential oil

- 5 drops of Lemon essential oil

- 5 drops of Rosemary essential oil

Massages

Cellulite Massage

One of these listed formulas is perfect to massage areas where cellulite is bothersome to you. Massage areas for at least 30 minutes. Keep the formulas on your skin for at least one hour after the massage.

Use 1-2 oz. of carrier oil with these essential oil blends. (Jojoba is awesome as a carrier oil).

- 8 drops of Litsea cubeba oil (this essential oil has a citrusy tang and is the botanical name of May Chang; a tree that is native to south China)

- 7 drops of Lemon essential oil

- 3 drops of Celery seed essential oil

- 2 drops of Balsam (Peru)

- 5 drops of Lime essential oil

- 4 drops of Cedar wood (recommends cedar wood from Texas, but that is your choice)

- 3 drops of Black pepper essential oil

- 8 drops of Cypress essential oil

Weight Loss Massage

Ingredients

- 2 0z. Sweet almond oil

- 5 drops of grapefruit, lemon or cypress essential oils.

Instructions

Mix oils together and pour into a dark, glass bottle. Put the lid on and shake or roll the bottle between your palms. This will mix the oils with the carrier.

Abdominal Massage

Massage the oil into your abdomen using large circles starting above your belly button and working outward toward the left side of your abdomen. Ideally, perform this massage daily, or at least five times weekly to obtain best results.

Chapter 3

DEPRESSION AND ANXIETY

If you are sad or just generally not feeling well, try natural depression remedies mailed with essential oils. Smell is often the pick me up you need. Aromatherapy home remedies for depression, anxiety, tension and unhappiness can help with that terrible feeling of not being where you want to be. Try aromatherapy and include it with other happy activities like exercise. Aromatherapy will not "cure" depression, but it will trigger positive responses by stimulating your body's limbic and endocrine systems. Try several blends and lone oils. You will quickly find what helps you feel better. I find that anything lemony or citrusy make me feel happier.

There are two types of depressions, one is situational and the other is clinical depression. When you are down and it is a situation causing your moods, there is always a way to "snap out of it." It might take some time, but it is possible to get over it and move one. Clinical depression is caused by a chemical imbalance in our brain. It is hard to snap out of it, but essent5ial oils can be vital in your fight against clinical depressions.

Researchers believe that the essential oils contain certain chemicals that activate aroma receptors in the nose connected to the area of the brain related to moods. If you are suffering from depression, there are certain oils that can bring about a sense of calm or elevate your mood.

Jasmine, sandalwood, clary sage, basil, ylang-ylang, bergamot, neroli, rose, lavender, lemon, geranium, and petigrain are a few essential oils that have been used to help with depression.

Clary sage essential oil is used in treating some types of depression, anxiety and insomnia.

Basil lifts anxiety and depression and can help lower fatigue.

Rose essential oil is wonderful for the entire nervous system and nervous disorders.

Ylang-ylang is a great relaxer. It also helps get rid of depression and helps with insomnia.

Sandalwood has a very nice sedative property good for treating depression and tension.

Lavender essential oil is perfect for nervous system disorders. It will help with depression, headaches, hypertension, insomnia, migraines, nervous tension and other stress related conditions.

Inhaling

Pour a teaspoon of coarse sea salt in a very small dark glass bottle. This is a mini aromatherapy inhaler and works wonders.

Irritable Depression

- 10 drops Bergamot essential oil

- 5 drops Grapefruit

- 4 drops Sweet Orange

- 1 drop Geranium essential oil

- 1 drop Ylang-Ylang essential oil

Grief-Related Depression

- 10 drops Rose Absolute or Rose Otto essential oil

- 4 drops Sandalwood essential oil

- 4 drops Neroli OR Petitgrain essential oil

Anxious Depression

- 8 drops Lavender essential oil

- 8 drops Grapefruit essential oil

- 2 drops Marjoram essential oil

- 1 drop Chamomile essential oil

- 1 drop Geranium essential oil

Depression/Guilt, relaxant

- 15 drops Geranium

- 5 drops Lavender

- 10 drops Bergamot

- Mix together. Use in a diffuser or as a massage. If using as a massage oil, add 3 tablespoons of carrier oil.

Guilt

- 20 drops Sandalwood

- 5 drops Roman Chamomile

- 5 drops Clary Sage

- Mix together. Use in a diffuser or as a massage. If using as a massage oil, add 3 tablespoons of carrier oil.

Mild Depression

- 4 drops Lemon

- 8 drops Coriander

- 4 drops Neroli

- 3 drops Ylang-Ylang

- 3 tablespoons Carrier Oil

- Mix together. Use in a diffuser or as a massage. If using as a massage oil, add 3 tablespoons of carrier oil.

Massage

Mood Uplifting Massage

- 5 drops Lemongrass

- 5 drops Geranium

- 3 drops Basil

- 2 drops Lime

- 1 tablespoon Carrier oil

- Massage oils into your upper chest, back of the neck and the shoulders.

Mood Elevation Mist Spray

- 50 drops Rosewood

- 35 drops Lemon

- 35 drops Melissa

- 30 drops Geranium

- 4 fluid ounces pure water

Banish Baby Blues

- 5 drops Angelica Root

- 8 drops Geranium

- 6 drops Bergamot

- Diffuse, sprinkle on a handkerchief, or use as a massage oil by adding 1 tablespoon of a high quality carrier oil

Chapter 4

HOMEMADE ALL PURPOSE CLEANER RECIPES

Save tons of money and feel good about your home cleaning products. Chemical cleaning products are dangerous and are linked with asthma, headaches, allergies, and eczema. Stop buying commercial cleaning products; get a life and make your own environmentally friendly and healthy cleaning products. Not only will you live an eco-friendly life, but it will cost you pennies instead of dollars to make your own cleaners.

One very nice all-purpose cleaner can be used anywhere. Use it to clean sinks, toilets, countertops, kid's rooms, playrooms and just about any room in the house. This cleaner is also awesome as dust aid or to the upholstery and dashboard of your car. Basically this cleaner will be awesome for anywhere you want to use it. Just a quickie note, don't use it on mirrors or windows. It will leave an oily residue. We will get to glass cleaners in just a bit.

Ingredients

1 teaspoon borax

1/4 cup white vinegar

2 cups of water

30 drops essential oil blend (see below)

Instructions

- Boil the water and pour into a bowl with a spout.

- Add borax and stir until dissolved.

- Add vinegar.

- Drop in essential oils.

Blend #1: Citrus Fruit Blend

- 3 parts of Lemon essential oil

- 1 part of Lavender essential oil

- 1 part Bergamot essential oil

Blend #2: Citrus Fruit Blend

- 4 part lime essential oil

- 2 parts Sweet orange essential oil

- 1 part Grapefruit essential oil

Blend #3: Herbal Blend

- 5 part Lavender essential oil

- 4 parts Rosemary essential oil

- 2 parts Eucalyptus essential oil

Blend #4: Flowery and Fresh Blend

- Equal part lavender and lemon essential oils.

- Add essential oils after your pour the cleaner into the spray bottle. Essential oils can "stick" to your measuring cup.

Window Cleaning Recipes

Super-Simple Vinegar Window Cleaning Recipe

- Mix 2/3 cup (170 ml) white vinegar with 1 1/3 cups (330ml) distilled water. Mix in 5 drops lemon or lavender essential oils in a spray bottle. Shake well and clean your mirrors and windows.

This recipe is really that simple. Vinegar is known as a natural cleaner and lemon essential oil is also known to cut grease and dirt. Try using crumpled up newspaper or a microfiber cloth with this spray. I have done an entire house using this recipe and crumpled newspaper. It works beautifully and shows now streaks when the sun shines through.

Heavy Duty Homemade Glass Cleaner Recipe

When doing your spring cleaning, use this window cleaner recipe. It is awesome!

Mix together 1 cup or 250ml each of water and white vinegar or vodka (a waste of good vodka!) Ad ¼ teaspoon (2ml) of liquid dishwashing soap in a spray bottle. Add 5 drops of lemon, tea tree or lavender essential oil. Shake well and go to town washing our windows.

Laundry Products

Homemade Laundry Soap

Purchase a clean gallon bucket for this homemade laundry soap. You might want to ask a restaurant for their empties, but you will need to clean it with hot water. (You can find 1 gallon buckets in dollar starts for a very low price).

Ingredients

- 4 cups hot boiled Water

- 1 natural Soap Bar

- 1 cup Washing Soda

- 1/4 cup Borax

- 30 drops Lavender essential oil

- 30 drops Lemon essential oil

- 30 drops Grapefruit OR Clove essential oil

Instructions

- Grate the soap bar using a cheese grater (or the type of grater used by pedicurists works well. I also like Ivory Soap).

- Mix the soap flakes and hot water in a large pan and stir over medium to low heat until the soap is melted.

- Add 2.5 gallon so very hot water to the five gallon bucketed. Add melted soap mixture, washing soda and borax. Stir until all the powder is dissolved.

- Fill the bucket with 2.5 more gallons of hot water. Cover and let the mixture sit overnight. The mixture will thicken.

- Don't despair if your dry laundry detergent is lumpy. My always does. I did what most people would do, I plunged my hands into the soap and squished the lumps. Worked really lovely and I had a great time squishing lumps of really awesome smelling soap.

- Well it really wasn't all that awesome smelling until I stirred the essential oils into the laundry soap mixture. Transfer the mixture to convenient jars or boxes.

- Shake or stir the mixture after each use to dissolve lumps that may have formed. Use 1 cup per load for top-loading machines and half a cup for front-loaders.

Do not mistake washing soda made from sodium carbonate with baking soda. You can find sodium carbonate in the laundry area of your grocery store. You can also purchase washing soda online.

Carpet Deodorizers and Scrubbers

Floor Cleaning Products

- You can use pine, sweet orange, peppermint, and eucalyptus and tea tree essential oils. There are different recipes and/or blends to add to your cleaning solutions. These work wonders for tile and laminate floors.

- Use the floor cleaner you regularly use and add 2part pine essential oil and 1 part cypress essential oil of a pine fresh blend. Use 2 parts sweet orange essential oil and 1part lemon essential oil for a fresh citrus smell and extra deodorizing powder. If you long for a minty fresh room, add equal parts of eucalyptus, peppermint and sweet orange essential oil to your cleaners.

Carpet Deodorizers and Scrubbers

- Combine essential oils with baking soda or other ecofriendly powders to make a scented powder for your carpet or for scrubbing counters, sinks, and other hard surfaces. You can either sprinkle the scrubbing powder on the surface of made a soft scrubber.

- Add these essential oils to your baking sodas and powders:

- Flowery sweet blend uses 2 part lavender essential oils and 1 part vanilla essential oil

- A flowery savory blend uses 2 parts lavender essential oil and 1part rosemary essential oil.

- Be a romantic and use equal part rose and geranium essential oils.

- Herbal lemon blend is nice and requires 2 part lemon essential oil, 1 part lemongrass essential oil and 1 part chamomile essential oil.

- There are many all-natural cleaning solutions using essential oils. Some essential oils kill bacteria and mold. They can be very strong so don't think more is better. One drop of peppermint oil is as potent as 30 cups of peppermint tea.

Chapter 5

MISCELLANEOUS CLEANING RECIPES AND USES

Have gunky combs and brushes that you need to clean?

- Fill a bottle with 1 1/2 cups of water, ½ cup distilled white vinegar, and 20 drops of tea tree, eucalyptus or lavender essential oil. Soak you combs and brushes for 30 minutes. Rinse and use with confidence.

- Scummy shower doors can be cleaned with just a few drop of lemon essential oil twice a month. The lemon oils will also protect shower doors from grimy buildup.

- If you have gum encrusted in clothing or on furniture or countertops, orange essential oils is perfect at removing this icky substance. Orange essential oil will not stain fabrics but rinse with water or launder immediately. Use a clean cloth or a cotton ball to apply.

- Cleaning toilets is an awful job. We call it the toxic waste job in our home. You can make this chore much easier by adding 2 teaspoons of tea tree oil and 2 cups of warm water to a spray bottle. Shake and spritz along the toilets inside rim, outside and on the floor. Let sit for about 30 minutes and then scrub. Tea tree disinfects, is antibacterial, and smells clean.

- A fun note: Add a few drops of a very scented essential oil on the inside of the toilet paper tube. When the paper is used and the tube unrolled, the scent will be released. Awesome bathroom deodorizer.

Herbal Disinfectant

A super disinfectant formula that's incredibly easy to make.

Ingredients

- 2 cups hot water

  10 drops thyme essential oil

  1/4 cup washing soda

Instructions

- Combine all ingredients in a spray bottle and shake well. Spray on surfaces and wipe clean with a damp cloth or sponge.

Citrus Dishwashing Blend

Dishwashing liquids have been designed to lure the consumer with their stimulating lemony scent. Their aromatic choice is more than an advertising gimmick; citrus oils are natural degreasers. It's the rest of the ingredients in these harsh detergents we are better off without.

Ingredients

- Liquid castile soap

  20 drops Lime essential oil

  10 drops Sweet orange essential oil

  5 drops Citrus seed extract

Instructions

- Fill a clean 22-ounce squirt bottle with castile soap (diluted according to Instructions if using concentrate). Add the essential oils and extract. Shake the bottle before each use. Add 1 to 2 tablespoons of liquid to dishwater and wash as usual.

Super-Easy Automatic Dishwasher Powder

Easy, cheap, smells awesome, and works! What else do you need?

Ingredients

- 1 cup Baking Soda

- 1 cup Borax

- 20 drops Lemon or Clove essential oil (or you can use 10 drops of each)

Instructions

- Combine the baking soda and the borax in a plastic container.

- Drop and stir in the essential oils.

- Cover and store in a cool, dark cupboard.

- Add 2 to 4 tablespoons homemade dishwasher detergent to your dishwasher's soap dispenser.

Liquid Dish Soap

Ingredients

- 1 cup Baking Soda

- 1 cup Borax

- 1 cup boiling Water

- 1 cup store-bought liquid dishwasher soap

- 10 drops Grapefruit essential oil

- 10 drops Lemon essential oil

- 10 drops Orange essential oil

Instructions

- Dissolve the baking soda and borax in the hot water.

- Stir in the liquid dishwasher detergent, then add the essential oils, mix well.

Sink Scrubber for Stains

Put this formula on the stain and leave for a few minutes. The scrub and rinse with vinegar and hot water. You will be surprised at the gorgeous clean sink you have.

Ingredients

- 1/4 cup washing soda

  1/4 cup baking soda

  8 drops rosemary, eucalyptus or tea tree essential oil

  3/4 cup vinegar for rinsing

Instructions

Combine washing soda, baking soda and essential oil in an airtight container and shake well to blend. Sprinkle a small amount into the sink and scrub with a damp sponge. Rinse the sink with vinegar, then with hot water.

Oven cleaning formula for baked on foods

If oven is not self-cleaning, and mine is not. I bought my range for looks rather than convenience. This formula is great. Baked-on grease and food splatters might require fine steel wool scrubbing on those areas. You can also use more salt.

Ingredients

- 1/2 cup salt

  1/4 cup washing soda

  1 box baking soda

  1/4 cup water

  3/4 cup white vinegar

  10 drops thyme essential oil

  10 drops lemon or lemongrass essential oil

(Remember that washing soda and baking soda are two completely different ingredients and you need them both for this recipe.)

Germs-Be-Gone Toilet Cleaner

Gunky toilets. This is an antibacterial spray cleaner formulated for cleaning the general surface areas of the toilet. Don't forget under, behind and on top of the seat.

Ingredients

- 2 cups water

  1/4 cup liquid castile soap

  1 tablespoon tea tree essential oil

  10 drops eucalyptus or peppermint essential oil

Instructions

- Combine all ingredients in a spray bottle and shake well. Spray on toilet surfaces and wipe clean with damp cloth or sponge.

Peppermint Foam Carpet Shampoo

I really like this for those areas that are particularly dirty; like high traffic areas.

Ingredients

- 3 cups water

  3/4 cup liquid castile soap

  10 drops peppermint essential oil

Instructions

Mix all ingredients in a blender. Rub foam into soiled areas with a damp sponge. Let dry thoroughly, then vacuum.

Awesome Kitchen Wipes

- Paper towels can get expensive; especially if you use them often. Instead of paper towels store multiple squares of cotton cloth in a container filled with 1 cup of water, 1 ounce liquid castile soap and 8 drops of your favorite essential oil (mine is lemon). You can also wash the clothes and return them to the jar for further use. Inexpensive and very eco-friendly.

Tough Cleaning Jobs and Essential Oils

- Greasy dishes will come clean if you add 1/2 cup vinegar and/or lemon essential oil to dishwater.

- Baked on food in pots and pans are a bother. Immediately after cooking, add some baking soda (and water) to the dirty dish and wait 15 minutes. If the pan has cooled, boil a solution of 1 cup water, 5 drops cedar or other essential oil, and 3 tablespoons baking soda directly in the pot or pan. Allow mixture to stand until food can be scraped off easily.

Notes on Cleaning with Essential Oils

Use only pure and undiluted essential oils. Any other type will not be affective. Pure and quality essential oils come in blue or brown dark glass bottles. If you store your essential oils way from heat and direct sunlight they can retain their potency forever. Citrus oils are the one exception; they only last for up to one year.

But, you will have used your lemony essential oils long before the year is up.

When using essential oils in a recipe use only the amount called for. Essential oils are highly concentrated and adding more won't make your recipe super strong. Instead, it will increase the risk of skin irritation. Use caution when handling essential oils and do wear protective gloves. Don't let your children handle essential oils. Take very special care of food-related oil. Citrus oils smell awesome and a child might think that they are drinkable. Keep all blends and recipes away from pets and children just to be on the safe side.

Controlling Kitchen Pests

Even the cleanest of kitchens are susceptible to unwanted visitors. I remember once when I finished scrubbing my kitchen tiled floor (on my hands and knees!), I came back an hour later to find a parade of ants walking across the floor. Yuck! My first thought was to go and purchase chemical ant traps, but instead I used these essential recipe ideas. They worked wonders. No more ant parades.

Ants

- Wipe cabinets and countertops with a damp clean rag and 6 to 8 drops citronella or peppermint essential on the rag. Drop 3 to 5 drops of the same oil on windowsills, doorway cracks and in the corners of cabinets, and under the kitchen sink.

Silverfish, earwigs and Centipedes

- Peppermint, eucalyptus or citronella essential oils get rid of these unwanted pests. Drop up to three drops of eucalyptus, citronella or peppermint essential in areas that tend to be humid. These areas are basements, plumbing cabinets and garages.

Mice

- These nasty little creatures breed like crazy, so don't let them get a foot-hold in your home. Get a cat, or place sprigs of fresh peppermint between items in your cabinets. You can also make a solution using of 2 cups of water and 3 teaspoons of peppermint essential oil. Put it in a spray bottle and spray it wherever you find mouse droppings. You might also put cotton balls with peppermint essential oil on them place in corners and near areas where mice get in your house. (Just a tip, I put cotton balls with peppermint oil in my outdoor barbeque).

Bug Repellents

Witch hazel contains alcohol. If you look, however you can witch hazel that is contains only natural alcohol.

Ingredients

- 14 oz. glass bottle

- 4 0z Witch hazel or ½ cup of water and a pinch of salt

- 1 Drop of Citronella, lavender and cedar wood essential oils

Instructions

- Mix ingredients in 4 oz. glass spray bottle. Spray skin and clothes. Is a determent to mosquitos and biting flies.

Insect Repellents

What you are doing is finding essential oils that mosquitos and other flying and biting insects do not like. These oils don't mix with water so you need to add them to carrier oils or alcohol (vodka works well). Be careful not to go crazy with the drops of essential oils. These oils are potent and could cause skin irritation.

Ingredients

- Mix your repellent so that it contains 5 to 10% of essential oils and 10-20 parts carrier oil or alcohol.

- Oils that work well against mosquitos and other insects are:

- Cinnamon oil

- Eucalyptus

- Citronella

- Castor

Best Cream Insect Repellent Ever

Sometimes kids don't like to be sprayed, and if you are a crazy sprayer you may get the repellent in eyes and sensitive areas of the skin. Use a cream repellent made with essential oils. It is very effective, safe, and smells good.

Ingredients

- 2 to 2 ½ tablespoons emulsifying wax

- ½ teaspoon stearic acid (this is a plant based stabilizer)

- 1/3 cup grapeseed oil

- ½ cup of distilled water or you can use lavender floral water.

- 1 teaspoon of vitamin E (open up a capsule if you need).

- 10 drops of Grapefruit seed extract (this is a natural preservative)

- 10 drops of Citronella essential oil

- 10 drops of Lemon Eucalyptus essential oil

- 10 drops of Lemongrass essential oil

Instructions

- Stir the oils, emulsifying wax and stearic acid in the top of a double boiler. Warm slowly over low heat until the wax is melted. Remove from heat and pour in vitamin E.

- In a different pot, gently warm the water/hydrosol until lukewarm.

- Pour the water into the oil mixture. Stir constantly with a wire whisk until the mixture is thick and cream-colored. Cool slightly.

- Stir in the essential oils and the grapefruit seed extract.

- Pour the bug repellent lotion into a clean and sterilized 8 oz. dark glass bottle. Allow the mixture to cool before putting on a lid.

- Shake the bottle occasionally as the lotion cools. This will prevent the ingredients from separating.

- Store in a cool, dark place.

Chapter 6

OTHER INTERESTING USES
FOR ESSENTIAL OILS

Everyday ills can be handled by essential oils. They are natural and will not cause chemical harm to anyone in your family.

- Warts can be healed by applying 1 drop of oregano to the wart. You may have to dilute oregano for if you have sensitive skin. Layer 1 drop of lemon and 1 drop of peppermint to the wart. Cover with a band aid. Use this recipe this at least twice a day until the wart disappears.

- All children have nightmares, and they just need a little love and monster spray to keep the nightmares away. Make your monster spray by adding 1 cup of distilled water into a fine-mist spray bottle. Add 5 drops of lavender oil. Let your child spray away the monsters. Not only will the monster leave, but the calming properties of lavender oil will help your child go back to sleep.

- Cuts, stings, bruises and burns can be helped by the application of 1 drop of lavender directly to the injury, sting or bruise. Cover with a cool damp cloths. You a repeat this every 20 minutes until the pain is reduce.

Mood and Stress + Germ Killers

Lavender 'n Lemon

- Equal parts lavender and lemon essential oils. Use 15 drops of lavender and 15 drops of lemon essential oils in water. Mix in a spray bottle. This is an all-purpose cleaning spray.

Mint Refresher

- Awesome for use as a glass cleaner and the spray keeps the room smelling sweet.

- Equal part of eucalyptus, peppermint and orange essential oils. Ten drops for an all-purpose spray or a drop of each essential oil for the glass cleaner.

Spice Splash

- 10 drops of Cinnamon

- 10 drops of Clove

- 10 drops of Lavender or Orange essential oils

This is awesome for scrubbing your bathtub.

Of course put in a water or alcohol carrier.

Guide to Purchasing Essential Oils

Where do you purchase therapeutic or pure essential oils? The answer depends on:

What are you using the essential oil for? If you are using essential oils to make something fragrant like a candle you do need fragrance or food grade oils. These are inexpensive oils and distilled using synthetic solvents. These types of oils are used by the perfume and manufacturing industry. Their purity is always questionable.

Using essential oils for your family, cleaning, and medical uses, you need to purchase 100% pure therapeutic grade oils. If you have a massage business or you do massages on the side, make sure the grade of essential oil you purchase is therapeutic and pure.

Therapeutic grade oils are required to meet stringent testing procedures as well as distillation measures. There are very few high quality essential oil suppliers in the world that produces these perfect oils because essential oils are very costly to produce. There are tons of companies that state their products are 100% pure.

Checkout how a company distills their essential oils. A reputable and responsible essential oil company is more concerned with producing quality products rather than the bottom line of its bank account. Thoroughly check out essential oil companies before you spend hundreds on inferior oils.

Read through the facts sections on websites and learn about therapeutic grade oils, distillation methods, and essential oil distiller sections. These will detail what to look for in an excellent essential oil distiller and the bottling and labeling requirements.

Read to discover as much as you can about the reputation of the company and if there is a wholesale program for frequent buyers. Once you have read through all the information you can find, you are now an educated consumer. Get ready and buy the essential oils you need.

References

http://www.realsimple.com/home-organizing/cleaning/all-natural-cleaning-solutions/essential-oils

http://www.motherearthliving.com/homemade-cleaners/natural-cleaning-recipes-zmhz12mazmel.aspx?PageId=2

http://mymerrymessylife.com/2012/09/homemade-natural-bug-repellent-recipe.html
http://www.easy-aromatherapy-recipes.com/

http://www.experience-essential-oils.com/

http://altmedicine.about.com/od/healthconditionsdisease/a/insect_repellents_oils.htm

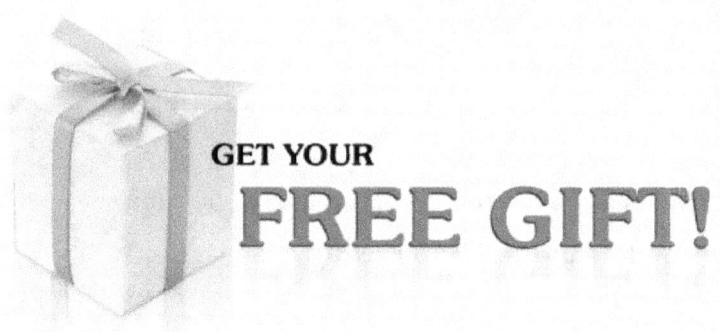

WAIT! BEFORE YOU CONTINUE – DO YOU LIKE FREE BOOKS?

My **FREE Gift** to You!! As a way to say **Thank You** for downloading my book, I'd like to offer you more **FREE BOOKS**! Each time we release a NEW book, we offer it first to a small number of people as a test–drive. Because of your commitment here in downloading my book, I'd love for you to be a part of this group. You can join easily here→ **http://joylouisbooks.com/**

Do You Enjoy **FREE BOOKS**? Do you like books that are Life Changing, Inspirational, Motivational and Informative? We **LOVE** sharing **FREE BOOKS** with people like you. It's easy to join just by clicking here→ http://joylouisbooks.com/

Check Out Joy's other book:
Essential Oils Guide for Beginners: The #1 Natural Resource for Weight Loss, Anti-Aging, Natural Cures, Healthy Lifestyles
See the book here:
http://www.amazon.com/Essential-Oils-Beginners-Anti-Aging-Aromatherapy-ebook/dp/B00UIEMIRG

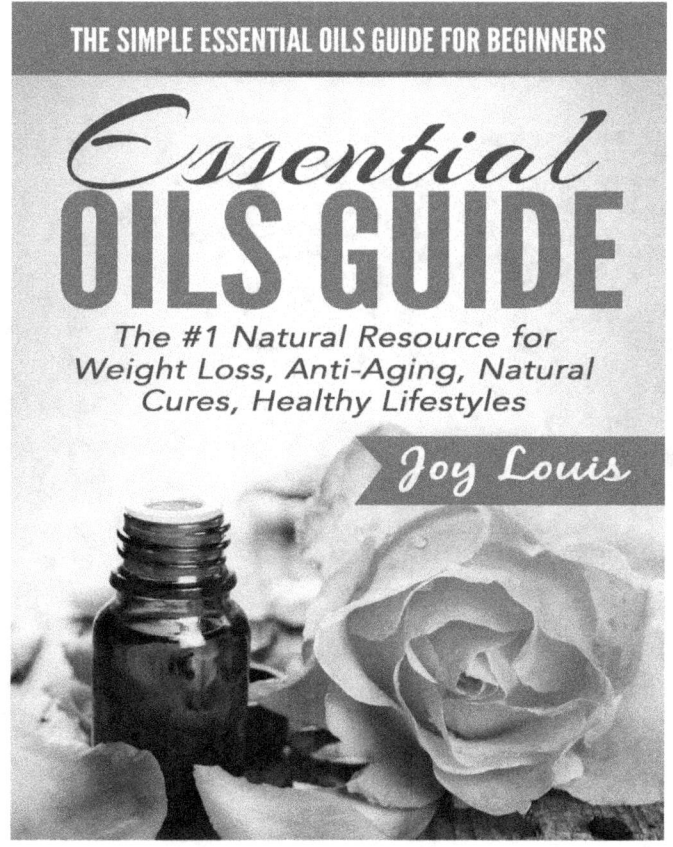

Conclusion

Thank you again for downloading this book!

I hope this book was able to help you to get excited about essential oils.

The next step is to look for more books on essential oils and natural living.

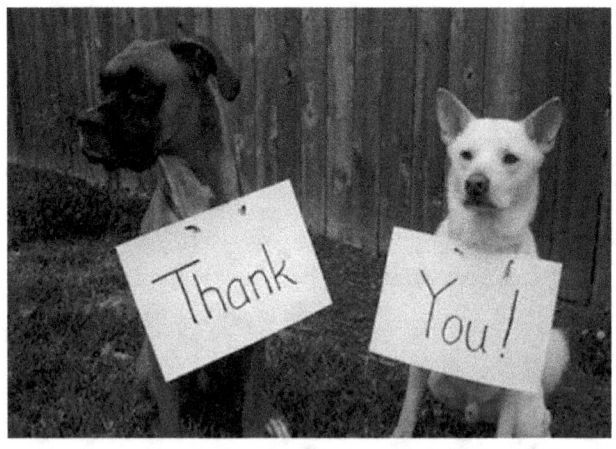

Finally, if you enjoyed this book, then I'd like to ask you for a favor, would you be kind enough to leave a review for this book on Amazon? It'd be greatly appreciated!

Click here to leave a review for this book on Amazon!

http://www.amazon.com/Essential-Oils-Beginners-Anti-Aging-Aromatherapy-ebook/dp/B00UIEMIRG